Robson Roose

Leprosy and it's Prevention

Illustrated by Norwegian Experience

Robson Roose

Leprosy and it's Prevention
Illustrated by Norwegian Experience

ISBN/EAN: 9783744693110

Printed in Europe, USA, Canada, Australia, Japan

Cover: Foto ©ninafisch / pixelio.de

More available books at **www.hansebooks.com**

LEPROSY

AND ITS PREVENTION

As Illustrated by Norwegian Experience

BY

ROBSON ROOSE, M.D., LL.D., F.C.S.

FELLOW OF THE ROYAL COLLEGE OF PHYSICIANS IN EDINBURGH, AUTHOR OF
"GOUT, AND ITS RELATIONS TO DISEASES OF THE LIVER AND KIDNEYS,"
"NERVE PROSTRATION AND OTHER FUNCTIONAL DISORDERS OF
DAILY LIFE," "INFECTION AND DISINFECTION," ETC., ETC.

LONDON

H. K. LEWIS, 136, GOWER STREET

1890

PREFACE.

During several visits to Norway, in recent years, I have had many opportunities of observing cases of leprosy, and of studying the forms and clinical features of the disease as it appears in that country. I have noticed, with deep satisfaction, the steady diminution in the number of cases, as shown by trustworthy statistics, and I have made inquiry into the causes which have produced so desirable a result. The little work, which I now offer to the profession, contains many facts which came under my notice when prosecuting these investigations; and I take this opportunity of thanking several Norwegian physicians (especially Dr. Kaurin, of Molde) for their courtesy and kind assistance, and for the information they readily afforded me. I do not, of course, profess to have given a complete account of leprosy; I have narrated its history and symptoms, but my especial object has been to point out the manner in which its spread may be arrested, and to invite attention to the lessons to be drawn from recent experience in Norway. I would advise those of my readers who are anxious to obtain full information on the subject of leprosy, to consult Dr. Leloir's magnificent *Traité Pratique et Théorique de la Lèpre*.

45, Hill Street,
    Berkeley Square, W.
        November, 1889.

CONTENTS.

CHAPTER I.

PAGE

HISTORY AND PRESENT DISTRIBUTION OF LEPROSY ... 1

CHAPTER II.

THE FORMS AND SYMPTOMS OF LEPROSY 23

CHAPTER III.

MORBID ANATOMY AND CAUSATION OF LEPROSY 47

CHAPTER IV.

THE TREATMENT AND PREVENTION OF LEPROSY ... 75

ERRATUM.

Page 11, line 19, *for* "one-fifth" *read* "one-fifteenth."

LEPROSY,

AND ITS PREVENTION.

CHAPTER I.

HISTORY AND PRESENT DISTRIBUTION OF LEPROSY.

LEPROSY is a chronic disease, distinguished anatomically by the formation of tuberous growths in the tissues. Its external manifestations are local anæsthesia, maculæ, thickening, and various alterations in the colour of the skin, pemphigus, the development of nodes or tubers, ulceration, febrile attacks, loss of portions of the extremities, atrophy of muscles, destruction of parts of the face, and especially of the nose, mouth, and larynx. Death occurs from marasmus, suffocation, syncope, or coma, or from intercurrent disorders.

Much confusion has arisen with regard to the disease, owing to the variety in the names by which it has been designated. The term "lepra" was first applied by Hippocrates and others to the complaint which is now named "psoriasis." When true leprosy became known, the terms "leontiasis" and "elephantiasis" were made use of to describe it. The latter name, however, was afterwards applied to the complaint now known as "Barbadoes leg;" while "lepra" was held to signify true leprosy. Hence it came to pass that very different diseases were described under the same name. We now speak of Elephantiasis Græcorum, or true leprosy (equivalent to lepra Arabum) and Elephantiasis Arabum (equivalent to "Barbadoes leg").

The earliest accounts that we possess of the disease known as "Leprosy" are to be found in the Books of Moses. It would appear that the Israelites, either while sojourning in Egypt, or during their wanderings in the desert, were attacked by a disease of so serious a character as to require the most severe and minute regulations in order to prevent its universal spread. Dr. Kalisch, in his excellent commentary on the Old Testament, states that in old traditions leprosy and other contagious disorders were not unfrequently represented as having really caused the expulsion of the Israelites from Egypt. Moses, however, attributes the Exodus to a very different cause, and his version of the case is generally accepted. It is enough for our present purpose to recognize the facts that leprosy was the most disastrous of the various diseases endemic among the ancient Hebrews; that it clung to them throughout their history, and that in all probability it first became known to them during their stay in Egypt. The endemic character which the disease acquired is shown by its prevalence during the epochs intermediate between the Exodus and the Assyrian, Babylonian and Persian periods, and that it prevailed at much later periods is shown by the number of miracles performed by Christ upon persons described as lepers. Whether the leprosy of the Bible was exactly identical with the disease of the present day is a question upon which much controversy has arisen; Dr. Kalisch states that the so-called "white leprosy" (which includes the anæsthetic and the tuberous forms) is equivalent to the *lepra Mosaica* or *Hebraeorum*, while elephantiasis, first and mainly attacking the feet, is probably meant and described in the Book of Job. Sir Risdon Bennett, in his little work on *The Diseases of the Bible*, states that there is no sufficient evidence that elephantiasis (true leprosy) is denoted in any of the accounts to be found in the Mosaic records. Perhaps the difficulty may be solved by supposing that the "leprosy" of the

Bible comprehended not only the disease as we see it at present, but other cutaneous affections more or less similar in appearance.

For many centuries after the time of Moses, Egypt was regarded as *the* home of the disease; but there is evidence to the effect that leprosy was known in India in the fourteenth or fifteenth century B.C. Some 800 years later, we learn that the Persians were afflicted with a complaint which was probably leprosy; isolation and expulsion of the sufferers were the simple measures they adopted. In process of time the disease was heard of in Europe, Greece being the country that was first invaded. It spread thence to Italy, having probably been conveyed thither by Pompey's troops. In the last century B.C. leprosy became established in the Roman Empire.

The spread of the disease throughout Europe is easily accounted for; wherever the Roman arms were carried, leprosy would necessarily follow. Military operations are especially favourable to the spread of contagious diseases. Many striking proofs of this statement are afforded by the history of syphilis, between which and leprosy not a few similarities exist. As a result of military invasions, not only is the diffusion of contagia increased and accelerated, but the gravity of the symptoms is liable to be much aggravated by the circumstances attendant upon prolonged and severe campaigns. The Romans doubtless conveyed the germs of the disease to Spain, France, and Germany, and although there are no records which enable us to trace its progress in Europe during several hundreds of years afterwards, the steps that were taken to check its spread in the seventh and following centuries sufficiently indicate the alarming frequency of the disease and the terrible character it had assumed.

We learn from Virchow's researches that in the early part of the seventh century, leper asylums existed in Italy and Switzerland, and at Metz, Verdun, Maestricht, etc. In 757 the Frankish King Pepin, and Charlemagne in 789, enacted laws with regard to the marriage of lepers. Dr. Hirsch's investigations show that leper hospitals were established in the Frankish kingdom in the eighth and ninth centuries; in Ireland in the year 869; in Spain in 1007; in England in the eleventh century; in Scotland and the Netherlands in the twelfth, and in Norway in the thirteenth century.

During and after the Crusades, leprosy spread with extraordinary rapidity, and excited the greatest alarm among those who witnessed its ravages. Leper hospitals were to be found in every part of Europe. It is estimated that in the twelfth century there were 2,000 such hospitals in France alone, and 19,000 in the whole of Christendom. It seemed as though an altogether new plague had been sent to punish mankind. Indeed, some historians have asserted that the leprosy of the Middle Ages was a newly-introduced disease, brought for the first time from the East by those who returned from the Crusades. As a matter of fact, however, the earliest date at which any of the Crusaders retraced their steps westwards was 1098, and there is abundant evidence to show that several leper hospitals were founded before that period. One of these institutions was established in England by Lanfranc, who died in 1089. Cases of leprosy of a very severe type were doubtless frequent among the returning Crusaders, and an extremely virulent form thus became rapidly superadded to the disease already existing in the various countries of Europe. The history of this spread of leprosy after the importation of new cases resembles that of the great epidemic of syphilis towards the end of the fifteenth century. So virulent were the symptoms of this outbreak that the disease was erroneously supposed to have made for the first time its appearance in Europe.

In some highly interesting articles which appeared in the *Edinburgh Medical and Surgical Journals* for 1841-42, the late Sir J. Simpson has given an exhaustive account of leprosy and leper houses in England, Scotland, and Ireland, from the earliest times. He points out that these hospitals were simply receptacles for infected persons, and not medical institutions, for the disease was regarded as absolutely incurable. The patients were engaged in religious duties, and subjected to hard discipline. They appear, however, to have been well cared for; they were supplied with good diet and clothing, and sanitary rules of various kinds were strictly enforced. In England, between 1100 and 1472, no fewer than 112 such hospitals were built and richly endowed. Some were founded by the wealthy and noble after they had themselves become victims of the malady. The largest leper hospital in England was at Sherburne, about three miles from Durham; it was built by Bishop Pudsey in 1181. At this hospital, we are told, refractory lepers were sometimes chastised with the birch "modo scholarium." Lepers, by English law, were classed as idiots or insane persons; they could not inherit any property, and were in fact regarded as though already dead. The Church performed burial rites over a leper on his admission into hospital; he was clothed, and in all respects treated as a corpse *in foro ecclesiæ.* Sir J. Simpson tells us that in France not many decades ago, the ritual still contained the office for the separation of the leper from the living. The ceremony must have been a painful one to the miserable sufferer; its final act was terribly significant. A shovelful of earth was thrown upon the leper!

The first notice of leprosy in Ireland is said to date from 432. There is a legend to the effect that St. Patrick maintained a certain leper in his house and washed the sores with his own hand. It is certain that the disease was very prevalent in later times. It was ascribed to the constant use of raw meat by the natives, and likewise to their foul gluttony "in the excessive devouring of unwholesome salmon." The complaint is said to have disappeared from Ireland when the English made laws against taking salmon out of season. There were at one period 18 leper hospitals in Ireland.

Leprosy was prevalent in Scotland in early times, though not to the same extent as in the adjacent countries. A hospital was founded in Glasgow, in 1350, and another in Edinburgh in 1584. The latter was pulled down in 1657.

The time at which leprosy practically disappeared from the British Isles is a point of considerable interest in reference to the causation of the disease. It is certain that the malady became very rare during the reign of Henry VIII. Shakespeare uses the word "leperous" in the sense of "poisonous" (*Hamlet*, Act I., line 779), and it is curious to notice that he attributes the breaking out of a "vile and loathsome crust" over a "smooth body" to the "leperous distilment" poured into the ears. Milton, in his description of the lazar-house in the eleventh book of the *Paradise Lost*, does not mention leprosy as an example of "maladies of ghastly spasm or racking torture," though he had doubtless often heard of the ravages of the disease. After the disappearance of leprosy, the hospitals became filled with cases of syphilis. Instances of the former disease were to be found in the northern islands of Scotland long after it had disappeared from the mainland. It was very general in Zetland in 1750, and Dr. Edmonstone saw a few cases in Scotland at the beginning of this century. In Ireland, the last recorded case was under treatment in St. Stephen's Hospital at Waterford in 1775.

Throughout Europe generally a progressive diminution of leprous cases took place towards the close of the fifteenth century. (The decline was most rapid in countries in which the condition of the people had been decidedly improved, and the strictest segregation of the lepers had been enforced.) There is also much probability in Dr. Hirsch's view that physicians had by that time learnt to distinguish between leprosy and syphilis, and that a more exact diagnosis of each disease had played a considerable part in reducing the number of leprosy cases. Still the fact remains, that for several centuries before the time in question leprosy had prevailed as an endemic disease throughout Europe, and that afterwards comparatively few cases were heard of, except in Norway and certain special districts. Dr. Leloir draws attention to the fact that in France the tuberous form seemed to pass away earlier and more rapidly than the anæsthetic variety.

The disappearance of the disease from Europe was followed by its introduction into the Western Hemisphere. It was doubtless conveyed thither by the European adventurers, and a much larger importation of leprous cases resulted from the arrival of the negroes. In later times the Chinese immigrants helped materially to spread the disease. Whenever the natives avoided contact with the strangers, as did the Indians of North America, they remained free from the disease. (Promiscuous intercourse, on the other hand, as in the case of the natives of Mexico, resulted in leprosy becoming endemic.)

One of the saddest instances of the introduction of leprosy among a people previously free from it is afforded by the history of the Sandwich Islanders. According to several authorities, the importation of leprosy into those otherwise fortunate Isles was due to the Chinese immigration in 1840. It would appear that at the present day nearly one-fifth of the inhabitants are affected with the disease.

Dr. Leloir points out that the history of leprosy clearly shows that this disease has always followed the movements of men, whether for warlike or commercial purposes, and that when a leprous race has come into contact with one previously unaffected, the spread of the disease has invariably followed. On the other hand, the people who hold aloof from the invaders escape from the plague, even if their condition as regards hygiene be as unfavourable as possible. Another fact deserves attention, viz., that the isolation of leprous patients by public authorities has always resulted in the diminution and eventual disappearance of the disease, and the rapidity of its subsidence has always been in direct proportion to the rigour with which the necessary measures were put in force. In subsequent pages, I shall cite several facts illustrating the effects of isolation.

The *geographical distribution* of leprosy at the present day is perhaps more important than even the history of the disease. Beginning with Europe, we find that the disease is endemic in a few districts, which are for the most part closely circumscribed. The most noted European centre of leprosy at the present time is the west coast of *Norway,* from Stavanger up to Tromsoe, most of the cases, as stated by Dr. Hirsch, belonging to the departments of Sondre and Nordre Berghus, which have been the head-quarters of the disease in that country from the earliest times. During a recent visit to Norway, and on another occasion (1887), I devoted some time to an examination of several leper hospitals, and through the courtesy of my friend Dr. Ed. Kaurin, of Molde, I obtained much interesting information with regard to leprosy in general, and particularly as to its prevalence in Norway. I found that the districts north of *Trondhjem*, and the neighbourhood of the *Sogne Fjord* were the principal centres of the disease, but that even in these districts there had been a decided diminution in the number of cases since 1879. The disease is, certainly, most prevalent along the seacoast. Dr. Kaurin informed me that in 1885 Norway contained about 1,195 lepers; he estimated their number at the present day to be from 1,000 to 1,100. In 1881 the number was about 400 in excess of the latter figure.

Since 1856, the number of lepers existing in Norway has been carefully registered by the authorities, and the results indicate a very gratifying diminution in the number of cases. In 1856 the number of lepers was reckoned at 2,113; up to 1869 there had been but little alteration, and some of the years show a slight increase. The diminution has proceeded without interruption since 1870, and thus it appears that the number has decreased by one-half in the course of thirty-three years. Dr. Hirsch's statistics indicate a still more remarkable diminution. He gives the number of lepers in Norway in 1856 as 2,847. The figures, however, which I have quoted above were taken from the Norwegian Official Statistics. In connection with these figures it is worthy of notice that the Molde hospital, built to accommodate 150 patients, now contains only 80. Dr. Leloir states that when visiting Norway in 1884 he found that the lepers entered and left the hospitals just as they pleased. They manufactured various articles, which were sold in the streets, and even mended boots and shoes. He saw at Bergen lepers standing in the market-place, offering eatables and other objects for sale. In the following year the Government decreed the absolute segregation of lepers. These enactments will be afterwards referred to.

In *Sweden*, a few years ago, about 100 cases of leprosy were said to exist; of these 86 were to be found in a small district in Gefleborg. *Iceland* probably contains about the same number. The condition of the remaining countries of Europe may be described in a few words. Cases exist, but are very rare, in *Austria-Hungary;* in *Russia* they are somewhat frequent on the shores of the Baltic, in Finland, in the Crimea, and among the Cossacks of the Ural. Leprosy is common in the Caucasus and in the delta of the Volga. In *Turkey,* there are small centres of the disease in Thessaly and Macedonia and in Crete (3·6 per 1,000). In *Greece,* there are a few cases on the mainland, and many lepers (about 300) are to be found in the islands of the Egean Archipelago. In *Italy,* there are several small centres of leprosy; one on the gulf of Genoa, and another near Commachio on the Adriatic coast. Sicily is another infected spot; it is said to contain about 100 lepers. In *France,* isolated cases are to be found near the mouths of the Rhone, in Provence along the shores of the Mediterranean and in parts of the Riviera. Dr. Leloir says that leprosy is perpetuating itself in these districts, and that new cases constantly crop up among persons born of healthy parents. In *Spain,* lepers are to be found in several provinces, and especially in Catalonia, Valencia, Andalusia, Galicia, Asturia, and

Granada. In *Portugal*, the disease is somewhat common, cases being especially frequent in Estramadura, Beira, Algarva, and in the mountainous district of Lafoës.

With regard to Europe, the general assertion holds good that, except in Norway, no attempt is made to prevent the spread of the disease.

Of all the countries which make up the continent of Asia, not one enjoys exemption from leprosy. In *Persia, China, Hindostan, Ceylon,* and *Indo-China*, the number of lepers must be simply enormous; *Hindostan* alone is said to contain a quarter of a million. In *China* and *Burmah* there are more lepers than can be found on the remainder of the earth's surface. Leper hospitals are as common in China as they were in England in the fifteenth century; they are always full, but their number is altogether insufficient. Near Canton there are two leper villages containing, perhaps, 1,800 inhabitants, and according to another statement there are 900 patients in hospitals within the city. In *Japan*, the disease is very prevalent, and widely diffused. We have, as might be expected, much trustworthy information with regard to the disease as seen in British India; no part is altogether free from leprosy, but the prevalence varies greatly in different districts. The disease is especially common in the hilly country of Kumaon, in Burdwan (Lower Bengal) and in certain parts of the Deccan. Hirsch states that in 1872 there were in the three Presidencies (Bengal, Madras, and Bombay) 99,073 lepers in a population of about 183 millions, the proportion to the population in the most leprous districts varying from 19 to 41 per 10,000. It may be regarded as certain that these numbers fail to denote the prevalence of the disease at the present day. As stated above, there is every reason to believe that the actual number of lepers in British India is not far short of a quarter of a million, and that the disease is steadily on the increase. Leprosy is common in *Arabia* and *Syria ;* Dr. Kalisch states that a colony of lepers is still to be found before the Zion gate of Jerusalem; they inhabit about 100 little huts.

The statement that no attempts are made to check the spread of the disease may be applied to every country in Asia. British India is, unfortunately, no exception to this rule. A few leper asylums certainly exist; but there is no compulsory isolation of the patients.

The condition of *Africa* as regards the prevalence of leprosy much resembles that of Asia. With the possible exceptions of *Tripoli* and *Tunis*, the disease is everywhere endemic. Throughout *Egypt* and *Abyssinia* the ravages of leprosy are everywhere visible; in *Morocco, Senegambia,* and down the *West Coast* lepers are constantly to be met with. In the *Canary Islands*, not many years ago, the number of lepers was officially stated to be 600. At the *Cape*, as we have been informed by a recent writer in *Blackwood's Magazine*, not only is the disease terribly frequent, and of a very severe type, but the manner in which the sufferers are attended to is disgraceful to a British colony. There are, it is true, two leper hospitals; one at Robben Island, in Table Bay, and the other in a mountainous district a few days' journey from Cape Town. With regard to the former, the writer in *Blackwood* says: "Here the patients live a death— to coin an expression—comparatively uncared for, and certainly unwept." As elsewhere, no measures likely to be efficacious are taken to arrest the spread of the disease.

On the continent of *Australia,* Dr. Leloir states that the disease has commenced to show itself in New

South Wales and Victoria, as a result of Chinese and Indian immigration. It is comparatively unknown in South Australia, Western Australia, and Tasmania. In *New Zealand,* according to Dr. Hirsch, the disease was once prevalent among the natives, but has decreased very much in recent years, though perhaps only in proportion to the terrible depopulation of the native territory. In *Oceania* the disease has become endemic in the *Sandwich Islands.* Opinions differ as to the date and manner of its importation. According to Dr. Hillebrand, of Honolulu (letter to Mr. Macnamara, February, 1866) the disease was unknown in these islands before 1859, and, after close scrutiny, could not be traced back further than the year 1848. Soon after the character of the disease became recognized the natives described it by two words signifying "the Chinese disease." Dr. Hillebrand could not determine whether the name was derived from a belief in the Chinese origin of the disease, or whether the natives had merely learnt from the Chinese immigrants that the complaint was common in China. At the present time there are about 1,400 lepers in the Sandwich Islands; of these about 750 are in the asylums on the island of Molokai (for ever hallowed by the life and death of Father Damien), and some 600 scattered about through the other islands.

It remains to add a few words with regard to the prevalence of leprosy in the Western Hemisphere. There are at the present time (*Medical News,* New York, June 22, 1889) many more lepers in the *United States* than at any previous period, the cases met with being nearly all imported from Norway and China. Their total number has been placed at 250, but this estimate is believed to be too small. The cases are most frequent in Minnesota, Wisconsin, and Michigan, at San Francisco, and throughout California and Oregon. In New Orleans there are no fewer than 42 known cases. In *Canada*, Norwegian immigrants are said to be responsible for the introduction of leprosy into New Brunswick, in the two counties of Gloucester and Northumberland, on the shores of the Gulf of St. Lawrence. In 1885 the Hawaiian Government requested the authorities of New Brunswick to supply information on certain points connected with leprosy as seen in their districts. The questions and answers have been published as a State paper, and contain much interesting and valuable information; they will be referred to in subsequent pages. In

Mexico and *Brazil* leprosy is very common, scarcely any district being exempt. The cases are especially frequent in and about Bahia, Rio de Janeiro, and Pernambuco; there are several large leper hospitals in Brazil. The disease is more or less prevalent throughout the States of *Central America*. In the *West Indies* leprosy is endemic in many of the islands. In *Trinidad*, with a population of 180,000, there are more than 480 lepers; in *Jamaica* (440,000) there were, not many years ago, about 800 lepers. Measures taken for the segregation of the diseased would appear to be of a very feeble character.

The following are some of the conclusions drawn by Dr. Leloir from a study of the geographical distribution of leprosy:—

"It is evident that the disease may develop itself in many and diverse climates, *e.g.*, in Iceland and Norway on the one hand, in the West Indies and Bengal on the other. It occurs both in hyperborean and in tropical regions, on the sea-coast, and on the elevated plateaux of the Himalayas, the Caucasus, and Mexico; its ravages are witnessed in mountainous countries, in dry and airy localities, and in low, damp, and marshy districts. It is difficult to determine whether climatic conditions exercise any influence upon the spread of the disease.

"All branches of the human race are liable to suffer from leprosy. The infected races may be classed in the following order, according to the degree in which the disease prevails among them: (1) the xanthous or yellowish-brown race; (2) the black; (3) the white; and (4) the red race. Many of the Red Indian tribes of America are still free from the disease, because they have kept themselves aloof from infected races. The tuberous form prevails in Norway, Trinidad, Spain, Madeira, and the Sandwich Isles; the anæsthetic form is more frequent in Hindostan, in the Philippines, and in Guiana. The mixed or complete form appears to occur with almost equal frequency all over the world."

Other conclusions to be drawn from the geographical distribution of the disease will be mentioned with the remarks on its causation.

CHAPTER II.

THE FORMS AND SYMPTOMS OF LEPROSY.

LEPROSY appears in two principal forms; in other words, is capable of exhibiting two distinct groups of symptoms. In one form, the skin is the principal seat of the manifestations; in the other, the nerves are especially implicated. The terms *cutaneous* or *tuberous*, and *anæsthetic* or *nervous*, are respectively applied to express the difference in the symptoms. That the two varieties are not to be regarded as two distinct diseases is proved by the similarity of the pathological products discoverable in both of them. Moreover, the two forms often coexist, the symptoms of one having been followed by those of the other. Cases of this latter kind are described as *mixed* forms; in the majority, the nervous symptoms become super-added to the cutaneous lesions.

(1.) **The tuberous or tuberculous form.**—The development of the characteristic symptoms is *usually* preceded by certain phenomena of a more or less indefinite character, and resembling those which are premonitory of other infectious disorders. They exhibit, however, this peculiarity—they are often experienced at irregular intervals for months and even for years before the appearance of the cutaneous symptoms. Indications of dyspepsia; headache; giddiness; mental depression; general debility; somnolence; lassitude; epistaxis; cutaneous hyperæsthesia; profuse sweating; irregular febrile attacks and pains resembling neuralgia and rheumatism are the most common premonitory symptoms. The entire group is very rarely found in the same patient; as a general rule, the history of the case shows that some five or six have been experienced. Perhaps the most common premonitory symptoms are the neuralgic pains, the alterations in the cutaneous secretions, the hyperæsthesia, and the febrile movements. In exceptional cases, the prodromal symptoms are altogether absent. They almost invariably subside when the eruption appears, and the consequent relief felt by the patient is often very considerable.

The setting-in of the eruptive stage is marked by the appearance of deep-red spots or blotches on the face and extremities. These are slightly elevated and of various forms and sizes; they show themselves in crops at irregular intervals and are often tender and irritable. A few of them may disappear altogether, but as a rule they undergo changes in colour, and become brown from pigmentary deposit, or else peculiarly white and dull and more or less puckered or striated. The maculæ often extend at their margins and coalesce, and this change may be in progress while the centres are becoming white and depressed. In the course of time, these maculæ become the seat of the tubercles or nodules. The macular stage may be prolonged for months or even years.

The *tubercles* or *nodules* begin as minute growths in the cutis, and slowly increase in size. Some of them eventually become as large as a hen's egg, others resemble peas; union of the nodules results in the formation of large irregular masses. The growths are soft, or at least not very hard, smooth, shining, at first dusky-red or livid in colour, but becoming yellowish-brown or bronze-like. The skin between them is more or less infiltrated and discoloured; there is slight desquamation of the cuticle and consequent roughness. The growths are usually tender, but not decidedly painful; they are not particularly prone to ulceration, except as the result of injury.

In some instances, the nodules coalesce and become soft and yielding on pressure; the surface gives way and a serous fluid escapes, with ulceration and crust-formation as a subsequent stage. After remaining open for an indefinite time, some of these ulcers may heal, while fresh crops of tubercles are being developed on other parts of the surface. Sensation is more or less affected in the diseased parts; in some cases, the tenderness of the nodules is replaced by anæsthesia; in others, the parts become intensely painful, particularly at night. Cicatrices left by the ulcers are for the most part devoid of sensibility.

The leprous nodules may break out on almost any part of the body; but they have a special predilection for the face, hands, and feet. When the face is covered by tubercles in various stages, the aspect of the unfortunate patient is hideous to a degree. All traces of normal structure are obliterated; nodular prominences, irregular in form and often separated by deep furrows, are distributed over the surface; portions of skin, visible between them, are hypertrophied and rugose; the lips and alæ of the nose are enormously thickened and furrowed, the nose itself is broadened and flattened; the supra-orbital and frontal regions project; the hair of the eyebrows, the eyelashes, and beard are wanting; the upper eyelid is swollen and everted; the ears (especially the lobes) are enlarged and prominent. Enlargement of the lymphatic glands under the lower jaw is another marked feature and adds to the hideousness of the general aspect. As can well be supposed, the face eventually becomes quite devoid of expression; the muscles are powerless to cause any change; suffering, misery, and hopelessness are terribly evident, and a close resemblance is observable among all the sufferers. It is impossible for a visitor to a leper asylum to guess correctly the ages of such patients; a youth, affected as above described, looks like an old man. When the eyebrows are much enlarged and the swellings project over the eyes, the countenance bears some resemblance to that of a lion or other animal: hence the term *leontiasis* has been applied to the disease.

Not only the skin of the face, but the mucous membrane of the nose, mouth, pharynx, and larynx is liable to be invaded by the growths. In these parts, flattened nodules make their appearance and sooner or later become ulcerated and excessively painful. In the nose, crusts form and obstruct the passages;

in the mouth and throat, the ulcerations render swallowing both painful and difficult, while a similar process in the larynx gives a roughness to the patient's voice and often reduces it to a whisper. The patient's breath, and indeed his whole body, become horribly fœtid. Destruction of the cartilages of the nose and larynx is a further step in the process. Another mucous membrane, viz., the conjunctiva, is prone to be similarly affected. Yellow and dark pigmented deposits are dotted over the sclerotic portion, and gradually spread to the cornea, interfering with vision and perhaps becoming disintegrated and causing total blindness. Iritis, irido-cyclitis, and synechiæ are by no means unfrequent. So common are diseases of the eye among lepers that out of 60 of Dr. Kaurin's patients, 41 were thus affected and of these six were quite blind. Other symptoms, more or less frequently met with, are connected with the generative organs. In women affected with leprosy, menstruation often becomes irregular, and sterility is the rule, to which, however, there are many exceptions. In males, the testicles are a common seat of leprous growths, and atrophy of these organs is the general result.

The process of the deposition of nodules on other

parts of the body resembles that observed on the face. Their formation is followed by their enlargement and coalescence, until the affected parts are much increased in size and exhibit the prominences and furrows, and the livid or bronze discoloration characteristic of the disease. The mobility of the limbs, and especially of the hands, is much interfered with, and serious excoriations and ulcers are liable to result from the slightest injuries. Glandular enlargement is another marked feature; besides those already mentioned, the inguinal glands are often swollen and prominent. Certain internal organs, *e.g.*, the liver, spleen, and mesenteric glands, are also liable to be invaded.

Sooner or later the symptoms of the anæsthetic form of the disease are superadded to those just described. But before this addition takes place fresh crops of tubercles are wont to appear from time to time, their development being attended by marked febrile movement, with headache, depression, pains in the joints, etc. These symptoms subside after the eruption of the tubercles; but they often recur, at irregular intervals, in the absence of any fresh local manifestations. These febrile attacks tend still further to reduce the strength of the patient; sometimes they assume an intermittent form and closely resemble the paroxysms of ague. In one set of cases, the nervous symptoms become very gradually developed; some of the tubercles slowly disappear, while the anæsthesia advances. In another group, a lengthy interval exists between the subsidence of the tubercles and the first nervous manifestations.

The course of tubercular leprosy varies greatly; in some patients it may be described as *acute*, in others as *chronic*. According to Dr. Bidenkap, the mean duration of this form is assumed to be from eight to nine years, but it is often much more prolonged. If the nervous symptoms become especially marked, the tuberous growths may subside, and the progress of the disease is then generally retarded.

In answer to my inquiries as to the relative frequency of the two sets of symptoms, Dr. Kaurin informed me that 70 per cent. of his cases belonged to the tuberous variety, and the remaining 30 per cent. to the anæsthetic form. According to the same authority, the latter is increasing at the present time, while the tuberous form is diminishing in frequency. Further details on this subject will be given in subsequent pages.

(2.) **Nervous or Anæsthetic Leprosy** generally begins in a very insidious manner. There may or may not be such prodromal symptoms as articular pains, resembling those of rheumatism, in various parts; weariness after slight exertion, pain and tenderness along the course of certain nerves, especially the median, ulnar, and peroneal; loss of appetite, gastric derangement, etc. The symptoms which eventually supervene are those of neuritis, acute as well as chronic. In the first instance, there are evidences of irritation of sensory nerves, *e.g.*, hyperæsthesia, neuralgia, sensations of itching, tingling, formication, etc. Sooner or later the motor nerves become affected; the limbs tremble and the muscles twitch; motor and sensory paralysis then set in. Another set of symptoms, viz., an eruption resembling pemphigus, atrophy of muscles and bones, and changes in the cutaneous pigment, indicates disorder of trophic nerves.

The disorders of sensation constitute the most prominent symptom. At first the affected limb or part is not only painful, but reddened in patches, swollen and hot; a nerve may often be felt through the skin as a thick cord; pressure upon it causes an increase of pain and other abnormal sensations. These symptoms recur more or less frequently, and then gradually pass into the opposite condition of anæsthesia, which finally becomes complete. The capacity for receiving impressions of temperature, pressure, and locality is more or less impaired, and the conduction of all sensory impressions is considerably retarded. In the later stages, when cutaneous and muscular sensation is entirely abolished, injuries to the part are unfelt by the patient. The portions of the body most liable to be thus affected are the hands and forearms, feet and legs.

The trophic disorders are manifested in the skin, muscles, and bones. An eruption of pemphigus is one of the most curious and characteristic symptoms. The bullæ are rapidly developed; they contain a fluid which is at first clear and yellowish; some are very minute, others are several inches in diameter; after a few hours or days they burst, and either heal quickly, or lead to troublesome excoriations or ulcers. The cicatrices left by the latter are at first more or less pigmented, but gradually become white, shining, and depressed. The sores are comparatively painless, and are frequently neglected by the patients; in some spots, and especially under the heel, they may remain open for a long time and increase in depth and width. Similar large vesications frequently result from injuries; owing to the defect or absence of cutaneous sensibility, the patients unwittingly expose themselves to extremes of heat and cold. The pemphigus, on the other hand, appears to be due to the irritation of the nerve fibres by the leprous growths. When anæsthesia is complete, the vesicles are usually wanting. Pigmentary anomalies constitute another group of cutaneous disorders, and appear in two forms. In the first, there is abnormal deposit of pigment in various portions of the surface; in the second, the pigment disappears from different parts, which become faintly yellow or even quite white. In the latter case, the condition resembles leucoderma.

The trophic disorders of the muscles give rise to conspicuous malformations; atrophy is associated with complete loss of functional capacity. Just as the tubercles show a preference for those surfaces which are most exposed to the air, so the muscles most prone to be attacked are those of the hands, feet, and face. The adductor muscles of the thumb, the interosseous muscles, and those of the little finger first begin to waste, and the natural roundness of the outer and inner sides of the hand gradually disappears. The muscles supplied by the ulnar nerve are most severely affected. The thumb is extended, the palm becomes flattened, the first phalanges of the fingers are extended, while the second and third are flexed, the hand thus acquiring that peculiar shape to which the term *main-en-griffe* has been applied. Many other muscles of the hand and forearm, and sometimes those of the shoulder, are thus affected; those of the feet are less frequently attacked.

The muscles of expression, supplied by the facial nerve, are often invaded, the paralysis generally commencing to show itself in the orbiculares palpebrarum. Other mimic muscles are attacked, and the power of expression is much impaired. The tears fail to reach the puncta lachrymalia and flow over the lower lids; inability to close the eyes results in lesions of the cornea. The lower lip falls, and dribbling of the saliva adds to the repulsiveness of the patient's aspect. As time goes on, and the muscular atrophy in the arms and legs reaches an advanced stage, the utter helplessness of the patient is the striking feature.

Another group of phenomena, connected with the

osseous system, often makes its appearance in anæsthetic leprosy. As a result of ulceration about the hands and feet, the muscles and fasciæ are destroyed, and one or more bones may become carious. If such ulcers be neglected, destruction of the bone will certainly result, and if many phalanges be thus attacked, portions of the extremity, or even an entire hand, may be lost. Another process is sometimes observed in the phalanges and metacarpal and metatarsal bones. One of the phalanges is found to be swollen and bluish; the swelling gradually increases; the skin eventually gives way, and an open sore results, at the bottom of which dead bone is found. After a while the bone becomes loose and is detached, and the wound then heals. Sooner or later, another bone is similarly affected, and the process may go on almost indefinitely until but few of the bones are left. The mutilations thus caused are multiform to a degree, and when combined with the results of muscular atrophy cripple the patient in every possible manner. So prominent is this group of symptoms in many cases of anæsthetic leprosy, that it is often described as *lepra mutilans*, and regarded as a variety of the disease.

In the final stage of anæsthetic leprosy the patient is reduced to a most miserable condition. More or less of the surface of the body is completely insensitive, the condition being always intensely marked in the face, arms, and legs. Owing to paralysis and atrophy of the mimic muscles, expression is entirely lost; the face resembles that of a corpse; the lustreless, widely-opened eyes indicate abandonment of all hope.* The hands and feet are horribly mutilated and deformed; many muscles of the limbs are profoundly atrophied; the surface presents ulcers in various stages, and yielding copious and foul discharges; cadaverous emanations are given off from the patient's body. Always thirsty, but having little, if any, desire for food, racked by torturing pains, the sufferer drags on a miserable existence, utterly heedless of all that is going on around him, unable to feed himself, and perhaps even to move without assistance. He often falls into a condition of stupor, and regards with indifference the progressive mutilation of which

---

* In this form of leprosy the ophthalmic affections result from the paralysis of the facial, and possibly from the anæsthesia, due to implication of the fifth pair. Out of 32 Norwegian cases of anæsthetic leprosy 15 suffered from diseases of the eyes.

he is the subject. A state of complete fatuity often precedes the termination of his sufferings.

The symptoms of anæsthetic leprosy vary in different cases; their development obviously depends upon the intensity and localization of the process in the various nerves. In the tuberous form the nerves never entirely escape; in the anæsthetic, the invasion of these structures is both severe and early, and the nervous symptoms are far more prominent than any manifestations of the tuberous type, which may eventually be superadded. In both forms, however, the growths affecting the nerves are precisely identical, and hence there is abundant justification for regarding the various phases of the disease as results of the same pathological processes. Even in cases of the tuberous variety the superficial nerves are considerably enlarged. The connective-tissue sheath is filled with a firm albuminous material in which the fibres are imbedded. In the anæsthetic form the changes are far more decided. Throughout the greater part of their course the large nerve-trunks of the affected part are thickened so as to resemble spindles, while here and there well-defined swellings mark special deposits of leprous material. The nerve-trunks also exhibit various changes of colour; some are red, others reddish-yellow, and in advanced cases a brownish or even dark brown colour may be presented. The jelly-like mass in which they are imbedded is made up of small nucleated cells; it penetrates everywhere between the fibres, and eventually destroys them by compression, so as completely to abolish their conductile power. The process may be regarded as a chronic peripheral perineuritis, invading at the outset not entire nerve-trunks, but sets of fibres. This mode of invasion accounts for the isolated macular discolorations, and the apparently irregular distribution of the pemphigus, and of the anæsthetic areas.

The process which affects the nerves may doubtless extend to the great nerve-centres, but the implication of the latter is always secondary, and occurs at a somewhat late period. In the early stages, in cases in which death has occurred from some intercurrent disorder, congestion of the vertebral vessels, and particularly of the posterior spinal veins, constitutes all the change in the central organs that can be detected on examination. In later stages thickening and opacity of the membranes and copious exudation into the sub-arachnoid space have been noticed in several cases. At a still more advanced period a deposit of whitish gelatinous matter has been found on the internal surface of the spinal membranes, forming a layer of varying thickness, and in some cases producing, by its pressure, atrophy of the posterior columns. The cerebral nerves are liable to be similarly involved ; leprous deposits have been found in the Gasserian and ciliary ganglia, and indications of perineuritis affecting portions of the fifth, sixth, seventh, and eighth pairs of nerves have been noticed in a few cases. All the morbid changes found in the nervous system lead irresistibly to the conclusion that the process advances in a centripetal direction, and that the mutilations which result from a leprous affection of the nerves are essentially different from those which sometimes occur in connection with primary affections of the spinal cord.

It is a curious fact that the nerves of special sense are very rarely attacked. Sight, hearing, and the sense of smell are generally unimpaired, except as a result of local processes developing in the sense-organs. Taste is sometimes perverted or impaired, but the change is generally due to the condition of the tongue, which is often the seat of leprous deposits.

The mean duration of life in patients suffering from anæsthetic leprosy is said by Dr. Bidenkap to be about 18 years from the first appearance of the symptoms. It is, however, often difficult to determine the exact time of invasion, and the course of the symptoms as regards rapidity is greatly influenced by the conditions under which the patients live, and the care and treatment they receive.

Remissions in the course of the symptoms are very common. Sometimes the patient remains without any marked change for several years; in some cases, indeed, there is decided amelioration. A return of sensation to the anæsthetic parts has been occasionally noticed, and evidences of improvement in the general health are sometimes witnessed. So decided may the change become that the patient is looked upon as cured; so favourable a course is, however, extremely rare. Progressive depravation of health, chequered by occasional periods of quiescence, or even improvement of the symptoms is the ordinary picture which the disease presents. If, as often happens, the tuberous symptoms be superadded, the downward course always becomes more rapid.

It remains to say a few words on the so-called *mixed*

forms of leprosy. Such forms' are truly typical of the disease; a case of *purely* cutaneous or of *purely* nervous leprosy must be regarded as non-typical. We know that the virus exhibits a preference for the skin and certain mucous membranes, for the lymphatic glands, the nervous system, and certain viscera. If all these parts and tissues be invaded simultaneously or in very quick succession, the result is what Dr. Leloir calls *lèpre complète d'emblée*, or leprosy complete from the beginning. If the virus invade only the integument, glands, and viscera, the picture presented is that of tuberous leprosy. If, in such a case, the virus subsequently attack the nervous system, the blending of the new phenomena with the previous symptoms (which may, perhaps, diminish) results in the formation of a second group of mixed leprosy. A third group results whenever the virus, after having given rise to the phenomena of nervous leprosy, ultimately concentrates its action upon the integument, and produces nodules or tubercles.

It has been stated in a previous paragraph that the tuberous is more frequent than the anæsthetic form. Dr. Kaurin's reports of the Recknæs hospital (Molde) show that of 660 cases, 478 (72·4 per cent.) belonged to the former, and 182 (27·6 per cent.) to the latter class. No definite statement can be made as to the relative frequency of the two forms in other countries, and we can only speculate as to the reasons why the virus in one class of cases prefers to attack the skin, and in another the nerves.

Prognosis.—All that can be said with regard to the prognosis of leprosy may be summed up in a few words. The disease is practically incurable; in the vast majority of cases, the patient either succumbs to its effects, or dies from some intercurrent disease whose advent has been favoured by the condition to which he has been reduced. In tuberous cases, the mean duration of life is from eight to 12 years after the first manifestations. Sometimes the course is extraordinarily rapid, death occurring within a year. The anæsthetic form runs a slower course, the mean duration being perhaps 18 or 20 years in the absence of complications. In Norway I have seen several cases in which the disease had existed for over 20 years, and Dr. Leloir states that he has seen cases of anæsthetic leprosy, in which the malady had lasted for 25, 30, 40, and even 44 years! In the mixed class, those patients in whom the anæsthetic has supervened upon the tuberous form generally live far longer than others in whom the symptoms have pursued an opposite course. While confessing the general powerlessness of treatment to avert the fatal issue, there is no doubt but that the course of the disease may be decidedly retarded by the adoption of remedial measures of various kinds. These will be discussed in the chapter on Treatment.

A few words must be added with reference to the cases reported as "cured." In Dr. Kaurin's statistics, dealing with 596 cases and extending over a period of 24 years, only eight cases are thus recorded. These were doubtless instances of the anæsthetic form, in which the course of the symptoms was entirely arrested, and the manifestations of the disease underwent partial or complete retrogression.

A further examination of these statistics shows that marasmus or exhaustion is the most frequent condition (45·7 per cent.) which immediately leads to death. Next comes pulmonary tuberculosis (12 per cent.); next diarrhœa (10·8 per cent.), and next suffocation (9·3 per cent.). In 10 patients (out of 398 fatal cases) death was attributed to disease of the kidneys. It is obvious that the occurrence of complications of various kinds must greatly depend on the individual peculiarities and general circumstances of the patients, and to some extent upon the climatic conditions prevalent in the infected districts.

Diagnosis. — Owing to the great variety in the symptoms and the insidious manner in which they are often developed, the diagnosis of leprosy sometimes presents considerable difficulty. As a matter of course, the circumstances by which the patient is surrounded frequently aid in determining the nature of the complaint, even in the earliest stages. Where leprosy is endemic, even the prodromal symptoms will afford a clue to the real nature of the case. As a general rule, the anæsthetic form is less easily diagnosticated than the tuberous variety. Of the latter, the most characteristic features are the early eruption of tubercles about the face and hands; the swellings above the eyebrows with falling-off of their hair; the abnormal deposits and losses of pigment; the general brownish hue of the growths. The tubercles may, in some respects, resemble those of syphilis; but they are developed in a different manner, and are not subsequently covered with scales and crusts. Leprous ulcers likewise differ from those of syphilis. They are not serpiginous; their course is very slow and they often remain stationary. According to several authorities, syphilis may co-exist with leprosy; but the two diseases are quite distinct as regards their etiology. Lupus may resemble tubercular leprosy, but its manifestations are generally limited to smaller portions of the surface. The coexistence of large superficial infiltrations with transformations of colour in various spots is sufficient to distinguish leprosy from lupus.

Anæsthetic leprosy is characterized by the alterations of sensation in various parts, especially in the extremities; the painful swellings along the course of the nerves; the atrophy of the muscles and the vesicular eruptions. The deformities and mutilations are quite peculiar to the disease.

There is one affection, viz., *vitiligo* or *leucoderma*, the appearances of which somewhat resemble those of leprosy. Vitiligo is characterized by the development of white patches, with borders marked by a deposit of pigment. Small at first, they gradually increase in size, and by their coalescence produce discoloration of large areas, to which the intervening portions of normal (pigmented) skin offer a sharp contrast.

Sometimes, and without obvious cause, the discoloration rapidly spreads; sometimes the patches remain stationary for long periods. The hairs on the discoloured portions invariably become white; but neither the functions of the skin nor the patient's general health are in any way affected. In the opinion of Sir Risdon Bennett (already quoted), the leprosy of the Bible was really leucoderma. Whatever view be taken of this question, it is obvious that the two affections are in reality quite distinct from each other.

The morbid anatomy of leprosy will be briefly described in the next chapter.

CHAPTER III.

MORBID ANATOMY AND CAUSATION OF LEPROSY.

THE formations peculiar to leprosy consist of granulation or chronic inflammatory tissue, and belong to the class of infective growths. The so-called tubers or tubercles have their seat in the skin, subcutaneous tissue, mucous membranes, connective tissue of nerves, and in certain viscera. Diffuse infiltration also occurs. The leprous tissue consists of cells in various stages of development. In the cutaneous growths, these cells are found close beneath the epidermis; they infiltrate the corium and thence spread into the subcutaneous tissue. At first, they are identical with leucocytes; but eventually they become much larger, reaching perhaps four times their original size, though they usually preserve their shape. The tissue is greyish-white and slightly translucent; the cells are pale and nucleated, and sometimes contain vacuolar spaces; the large cells are regarded as characteristic of the leprous deposits. The nodules contain a copious network of blood-vessels. The tissue once formed, is very stable; the cutaneous growths may become disintegrated with consequent ulceration, but the latter is much more often the result of injury. Complete resolution of the growths is very rare; it occasionally results from fatty metamorphosis of the cells. Ulceration of leprous tissue deposited in mucous membranes is very frequent.

The leprous growths in the nerve-sheaths have a similar composition. As a result of the deposit, the nerve-fibres are much reduced in quantity, and hence we may account for the local anæsthesia and the muscular wasting. Moreover, the inflammation which accompanies the neoplasm causes the growth of new connective-tissue, which still further interferes with the functions and vitality of the nerves.

It is now generally considered that leprosy is due to the presence of a specific bacillus; the grounds upon which this opinion is based are thus stated by Prof. Neisser.*

1. The bacillus is met with in all leprous processes, in nearly all organs, generally within the cells con-

---

* See article in Ziemssen's "Handbook of Skin Diseases," and also papers on Leprosy in New Syd. Society's "Microparasites in Disease," p. 289, et. seq. (In the preparation of some portions of this chapter free use has been made of Prof. Neisser's essay.)

stituting the new formations, more rarely free in the tissues. In the recent state, and in unstained preparations, the bacilli are recognizable with difficulty; but easily after staining the tissue with most anilin colours. After staining, the covering should be rinsed in acidulated water; the preparations should then be dried and mounted in Canada balsam. By this method, only the lepra bacilli remain stained, other bacilli lose their colour. The micro-organisms thus rendered visible are extremely fine, slender rods; sometimes pointed or tapering at both ends, from $\frac{1}{2}$ to $\frac{3}{4}$ the diameter of a human red blood-corpuscle; their breadth is about one-fourth of their length; they are either straight or slightly bent. (See the illustration in the Frontispiece.) The bacilli therefore closely resemble those of tuberculosis; but they differ from the latter in their staining relations. Alkaline solutions are required for the bacilli of tuberculosis; while those of leprosy can be tinted also in neutral and acid solutions. The bacilli of leprosy are not coloured by anilin brown or by any yellow dyes. Instead of bacilli, small granular particles are sometimes found; these may be either spores or products of disintegration.

2. The bacillus is constantly present in all forms of leprosy, in all countries. The accuracy of this statement is now universally acknowledged.

3. In every case of leprosy, the bacilli are found in all the more recent new-formations in the skin, the mucous membranes, the cornea, the interstitial nervous connective tissue; also in the connective tissue of the spleen and liver; lastly, in the lymphatic glands, the testicles, and epididymis. The quantity found in these parts and organs corresponds with the degree of the affection. It is further stated that when the symptoms subside, and the new formations undergo partial absorption, the bacilli found therein exhibit corresponding signs of degeneration, become disintegrated, and either wholly or partially disappear.

In the *skin,* the bacilli are present both in the nodules and in the diffuse infiltrations. They are found almost exclusively in the large roundish cells described by Virchow. They may be either scattered throughout such cells, or may appear in small circumscribed accumulations. (See the illustration in the Frontispiece.) Sometimes two or three rods are attached to each other by their extremities; sometimes they are densely crowded together, so as to form a compact pile. The oldest layers of cells are immediately beneath the epidermis, and are often collected together so as to form large round accumulations. It seldom happens that free bacilli are found between the cells in the meshes of the connective tissue. The microscopical appearances in the *mucous membranes* closely correspond with those observed in the skin. Cells containing bacilli are found in the interlobular connective tissue of the *liver,* and even within the hepatic cells. Isolated foci, connected with large cells, have also been observed in the *spleen ;* the lymphatic glands exhibit extensive infiltrations in the peripheral zones, in which " blood-pigment, even macroscopically visible," has been found accumulated in large quantities. According to Dr. G. Thin the presence of bacilli in the blood-vessels has now been definitely ascertained.

The discovery of bacilli in leprous deposits around the *peripheral nerves* is a point of very great importance, and serves to explain many prominent symptoms. Neisser states that he failed to discover the bacilli in specimens taken from *advanced* cases; but that he found them in large cells, between the nerve-fibres and the bundles, in a specimen derived from a leprous patient who had succumbed to an intercurrent acute disease.

Finally, it would appear that bacilli have not as yet been discovered in the spinal cord or muscles, or in any of the epithelial tissues of the skin. They are said to take no part in producing the pemphigus and the affections of the bones and joints. These symptoms may all be regarded as *secondary,* and as due to the peripheral neuritis. Wherever the pemphigus appears, the skin is always more or less insensitive. The epidermis is declared to be inaccessible, both superficially and from below, to any invasion from the bacilli.

4. With regard to the origin of the lepra cells, it is sufficient to mention that two principal views have been advanced. Virchow considers that the fixed connective tissue cells are the mother cells of the growths; Neisser, on the other hand, alleging that Virchow's views can neither be proved nor disproved, maintains that the granulation cells are in reality emigrated white corpuscles of the blood and lymph. The same authority has experimentally demonstrated the manner in which these corpuscles develop into lepra-cells. He has also pointed out that bacilli may be found in every dry preparation of pus discharged

by ulcerating leprous nodules. "Cells in no way differing from ordinary pus-corpuscles are full of beautifully stained bacilli."

5. Every developmental phase of the lepra cell is accompanied by a corresponding state of the bacilli therein contained. As the cells become older and larger, the bacilli and their derivatives increase in number. At a later stage the bacilli are collected into large round agglomerations, sharply limited, and possessing a marked waxy lustre, but deeply stained by anilin. These masses represent the extreme phase of the bacillary infiltration of the cell-protoplasm. Changes likewise take place in the latter; vacuoles form, and large numbers of bacilli escape from the cells.

Prof. Neisser thus sums up the conclusions to be drawn from a consideration of the facts thus far enumerated:—

A specific bacillus, which has gained access into the tissues, is the exciting cause of the peculiar form and nature of the lepra cell: leprosy is, therefore, a bacterial disease. The bacilli are capable of cultivation on boiled egg-albumen, and on blood-serum with gelatin. It is difficult to find a species of animal appropriate for inoculation, and spontaneous leprosy has not hitherto been observed in animals. Neisser inoculated two dogs by introducing small leprous particles into the subcutaneous connective tissue, and the result was the production of local neoplasms histologically identical with the tubercles of leprosy, and containing many bacilli. No general symptoms were, however, exhibited.

6. Leprosy is a contagious and infectious disease. Many facts may be adduced in proof of this statement. In the first place, there are several examples of leprosy having been introduced into countries previously free from the disease, and of its rapid spread in the course of a few decades. The case of the Sandwich Isles has been already referred to. Fifty years ago, leprosy was unknown among the natives; at the present day, one-fifteenth of the aborigines are suffering from the disease. Another instance is afforded by the present condition of the Island of Trinidad. In 1805, there were three lepers among some 30,000 inhabitants; ten years ago, there were 860 patients among a population amounting to 120,000.

A very strong argument in favour of the contagiousness of leprosy is supplied by those instances in which persons who have immigrated into infected localities have been attacked by the disease. Father Damien's case is one of the strongest that can be adduced; the essential facts are few and simple. A young and healthy European went to a distant island in the Pacific, and after living and working among lepers for about ten years, began to show signs of the disease, from the effects of which he ultimately died. It is nothing to the purpose to say that we do not know how the virus gains access to the body, and the supposition that local telluric influences are sufficient to account for the origin of the disease can scarcely be regarded as tenable. As in the case of scarlet fever, measles, and small pox, it may be regarded as certain that a person never becomes leprous unless he has received the infection, either directly or indirectly, from a person suffering from the disease. Niemeyer's remarks with regard to measles, as the type of an infective disease, may be applied to leprosy. "It is sometimes asserted that the *first* case could not have been induced by infection, because at that time there was no such disease from which the patient could be infected; the inference is then drawn that if the disease developed spontaneously once, there is no reason for denying the possibility of its doing so again. Such reasoning is idle. We know nothing about the first development of measles," or (it may be added) of any infectious disease. We shall see by-and-bye that the most extraordinary ideas have been advanced as to the causation of leprosy.

In 1866 the Government of India published a well-known Report on the character and progress of leprosy in the East Indies, being answers to questions drawn up by the Royal College of Physicians, London. Similar information was derived from other parts of the world, and the College arrived at the conclusion that leprosy was not communicable by contact or proximity. It is worthy of note, however, that in 36 out of 107 medical reports from the East Indies, an opinion was expressed in favour of the communicability of the disease ; in 26 the question was regarded as an open one, while in 24 communicability was denied. The authors of several reports state that leprosy is contagious only in the ulcerative stages. It would probably be nearer the truth to say that the disease is particularly contagious when open sores exist. The discharges from these ulcers consist largely of pus, in the corpuscles of which, as already stated, bacilli can be easily demonstrated.

The opinion that leprosy can be propagated by direct contact has been recently fortified by the results of a very remarkable experiment. A murderer condemned to death in the Sandwich Islands was offered a commutation of his sentence (to imprisonment) on condition that he would allow himself to be inoculated with leprous matter. The offer was accepted by the man, and the operation was performed by Dr. Arning on November 5, 1885. In September, 1888, his condition was declared to be as follows:— Ears and forehead tubercular and considerably hypertrophied; face, nose and chin show flattened tubercular infiltration; face generally presents a leonine aspect. Hands puffed, proximal phalanges swollen, tips of forefinger and thumb of left hand ulcerated and anæsthetic. Body thickly marked with tubercles, of a yellowish brown colour, and presenting many patches of tubercular infiltration. Infiltrations on thighs as far down as the knees; legs quite smooth and even to the touch; feet œdematous, bluish. The seat of the inoculation, on upper third of outer aspect of left arm, shows a dark purplish scar, about $1\frac{1}{2}$ inches long by $1\frac{1}{2}$ inches wide, irregular in shape, keloid in aspect, dense and inelastic. Eyes affected with sclerotitis, muddy and injected. No signs of paralysis about muscles of face, orbiculares palpebrarum, hands or forearms. The President of the Board of Health and the Government Physician, Honolulu, who furnished this report, state in conclusion " It is our decided opinion that this man is a tubercular leper."

There can be no doubt as to the validity of this conclusion ; but the objection may be raised that the man was already leprous before the inoculation. It is impossible to prove that he was not thus affected ; but, considering all the circumstances of the case, there is little force in criticism of this nature. Other reported instances in which inoculation was performed without any results would seem to contradict the lesson to be drawn from the above-mentioned case. Dr. Leloir* records the following experiments:—Some 30 years ago, the venerable X— endeavouring to discover the cause of leprosy, and fully convinced that the disease was not contagious, inoculated himself with fragments of the tubercles, blood, pus, etc. After several repetitions of his experiments, with some amount of septic lymphangitis as the only result, he inoculated 20 other healthy persons, who

---

* "Traité Pratique et Théorique de la Lèpre," p. 237.

consented to be thus experimented upon. Lymphangitis alone was produced; there were no local manifestations in any way resembling those of leprosy. The patients were watched for many years, and all remained healthy. Dr. Profeta inoculated two women aged 25 and 31, and eight men, including himself and Dr. Camina, all having been made aware of the risk they were incurring. The result was the same in all the cases—an absence of any symptoms of leprosy.

Cases such as the above prove only that the virus of lepra is not always capable of being conveyed by inoculation from man to man. Various diseases evidently possess different degrees of contagiousness; there is every reason for believing that no one, unless already syphilitic, would escape infection, if inoculated with the discharge from a hard sore or the secretion of a condyloma. In the case of leprosy, other conditions may be necessary for the success of the inoculation, *e.g.*, a depraved state of health, due to one or more of a large number of causes; or, as Mr. Macnamara* expresses himself, "It may well be that

---

* *Leprosy a Communicable Disease*, 2nd Ed., 1889, p. 49. For many interesting facts bearing on this question, see Archdeacon Wright's little book "Leprosy an Imperial Danger."

the susceptibility to the development of the disease, even by contagion, is not universal."

That leprosy is to be classed among contagious disorders is shown, to some extent at least, by the resemblance its spread sometimes presents to that of diseases admittedly of this character. The case of the Sandwich Isles may be taken to show that leprosy introduced among a population previously free from its ravages is capable of spreading with alarming rapidity. In the Faroe Islands there have been several epidemics of measles; a very severe one in 1846 was the first that had occurred for 65 years. One case that had been introduced infected the attendants of the patient, and in the course of seven months some 6,000 persons, out of a population of 7,782, were attacked by the disease. The spread of syphilis and the frightful ravages committed by the disease in Polynesia, are analogous to the progress and to the characteristic features of leprosy, as seen at the present day in several of those islands.

Other considerations may be adduced in support of the view that leprosy is contagious. The disappearance of the disease under certain circumstances is a fact of this character. Neisser formulates the rule that the spread of leprosy stands in inverse relation to the measures to which the patients are subjected in the various localities. Wherever isolation is vigorously practised, and proper hygienic measures adopted, the spread of the disease is invariably arrested. The truth of the statement cannot be disputed, and the inference to be drawn from the fact is a very simple one. Too much attention cannot be directed to the Norwegian experience of the last 20 years. It is, of course, not denied that the spread of leprosy and the type which the disease assumes, are considerably influenced by such factors as climate, food, insanitary conditions, etc., and a few remarks will hereafter be made on these subjects. There is much reason for believing, with Prof. Neisser, that the virus of the leprosy seen in Europe is of a weaker quality than that of the disease as it prevails in the Sandwich Islands and many parts of the East. Pasteur and others have proved that some of the qualities of bacteria may undergo considerable modifications; their virulence, for example, may become considerably lessened, while their morphological qualities remain unchanged.

It remains to consider the various ways in which infection may take place. The contagious material may certainly be conveyed directly, and perhaps through the atmosphere and with food. It is not known whether the spores retain their vitality in dead bodies, as is the case with those of anthrax; but such a retention of power is not improbable. It would appear that the bacilli cannot penetrate through sound epidermis; some lesion of the protective layer is presumably necessary. In all probability, it is the spores that gain access to the organism, pass into the lymph-channels, thence into the lymphatic glands, and from these to various parts of the body. The parts most liable to be first infected are the face, the hands, the genital organs (as a result of sexual intercourse), the mouth, and the respiratory passages. The lymphatic vessels are the principal, if not the sole channel for the spread of the bacilli or their spores in the organism; microscopical investigations tend to show that the lymph-corpuscles take an active share in the conveyance of the bacilli.

Nothing definite is known as to the time required for the incubation of leprosy. There is not, as in the case of syphilis, any so-called primary lesion; when the symptoms are evident, the disease has, so to speak, become constitutional. Dr. Leloir cites one case, seen by himself in France, in which the period of incubation had extended to 14 years; Dr. Kaurin thinks that the ordinary period is from two to three years.

It is only fair to state that Dr. Hirsch and several other competent authorities deny the contagiousness of leprosy. Dr. Hirsch adduces the following facts as telling decisively against the doctrine in question :—

(1) The extremely narrow limitation of leprosy in certain centres, often very small, while there is free communication between their inhabitants and the neighbouring population, and where the sanitary conditions are such as would especially favour the conveyance of the disease sooner or later.

(2) At certain places, with a mixed population, the malady is confined to particular races or nationalities, notwithstanding unrestricted social intercourse throughout the community.

(3) The fact that in innumerable cases, the acquiring of leprosy by one member of a family has led to no other outbreaks of it in that family, even under very insanitary conditions. Both parents very rarely take it, and when this accident does occur, it may be referred to infection of both from a common source or to endemic influence.

(4) There has never been a case known in which the physicians or nurses of a leper-house have caught the disease (?).

(5) No case has come to light hitherto, in which the disease has spread from the leper-houses to residents outside.

(6) Among the many cases of leprosy in Europeans who had acquired the disease in leprous districts, not one has ever been the occasion of the disease spreading in the immediate neighbourhood.

One general remark may be made with regard to all these arguments, viz., that they are based upon a mass of information, which is nevertheless imperfect. The statement under No. 4 is contradicted by the cases of Father Damien, and of several Sisters of Mercy, and by the fact for which there is good authority that 10 per cent. of the attendants employed at Molokai become lepers. Even if the argument were true, it would by no means prove that leprosy is non-contagious. The nurses, dressers, and others, in Lock hospitals very rarely contract syphilis from the patients on whom they attend, and yet no one denies that syphilis is in the highest degree communicable. The limits I have assigned to myself in this little work will not permit of a longer discussion of this subject. Abundant evidence in favour of the contagiousness of leprosy may be found in Archdeacon Wright's and Mr. Macnamara's essays. I would repeat the observation, made in a former paragraph, that the malignancy of the virus of a contagious disease is not uniform under all circumstances. Moreover, we have learnt, from carefully-conducted experiments, that the same virus acts differently on various races of animals, *e.g.*, of mice or of sheep; it would therefore appear probable that similar differences may exist among different human races, and that even within the same race, the receptivity of the several individuals may not always be the same (Neisser).

The question as to whether leprosy can be transmitted from parents to offspring comes next for consideration. Dr. Kaurin informed me, a few months ago, that in the opinion of himself and his colleagues the disease was not thus transmitted. Dr. Hirsch, on the other hand, states that this method of the conveyance of leprosy cannot be questioned, and that "there is almost complete unanimity on this point among the observers of all times." The question may be divided into two parts, viz., whether the disease is inherited as such, or whether it is only a predisposition to be attacked that is thus transmitted. Statistics are, of course, the only means by the aid of which a decision can be arrived at. There are, however, two difficulties which must be borne in mind when dealing with statistics on this subject. In the first place, many of the observations have been made in parts of the world where accurate information as to the state of health of the lepers' ancestors could scarcely be obtained. Secondly, when the cases are collected in districts where the disease is endemic, the possibility is always present that some of the patients, even with a family history of leprosy, might have become affected through contagion. Dr. Hirsch mentions another objection against the doctrine of heredity, viz., the difficulty of accounting for the rapid extinction of the disease in such places as the Faröe Islands and certain districts in Sweden.

An affirmative answer to the question of heredity is, however, based on observations made in a considerable number of small, closely-circumscribed districts, with a tolerably fixed population, where the state of health of the various families may be traced through several generations. As examples of such places, Dr. Hirsch mentions various points on the coast of Provence, Commachio, Sicily, Southern Russia and the Caucasus, Greece, certain islands in the East Indian Archipelago, and New Brunswick. With regard to the last-named place, Dr. Taché, in the Report already quoted, states as follows: "The disease does not appear to me to be hereditary, that is, transmitted, *de toutes pièces*, from parents to offspring by procreation, or stored in the blood of individuals or generations, in its morbid nature and potential energy, without show of its presence. I doubt not, however, that the greater or less susceptibility to contract or acquire the distemper forms part of constitutional inheritance. . . . I know many instances where one member only of a family has been affected with leprosy, while all the other members remained free from any trace of it." Dr. Hirsch's conclusions are of a different character: " In all these places we do in fact find classical proofs that the disease clings to particular families as a consequence of continuous inheritance from generation to generation, and that the extension and multiplication of these small centres of disease is due to intermarriages among members of leprous families and of families who had been hitherto healthy."

Another excellent authority, Leloir (a firm believer in the contagiousness of leprosy), admits that the disease may be transmitted to the offspring, but thinks that many cases attributed to transmission are really due to contagion. His arguments in favour of the more frequent operation of the latter cause are as follows—

1. Leprosy is often observed among persons, none of whose ancestors have suffered from the disease.

2. Leprosy has been contracted in the colonies by Europeans, born of healthy parents, in non-infected countries, and with no family history of the complaint.

3. It is quite impossible to demonstrate hereditary predisposition in every case of leprosy, occurring in an infected district. In 107 cases, collected by Dr. Leloir, heredity could be traced only in 47 patients.

4. In some cases considered to be of hereditary origin, the parents appeared to be in good health when the child was born, though they subsequently became lepers.

5. The children of leprous parents do not always suffer from the disease. If such children live with their parents their chances of escape are very small; under opposite conditions, their chances are very

much increased, and especially if they are sent into a non-infected district.

6. The age at which the symptoms most often appear tends to contradict the theory of hereditary transmission. In the majority of patients born and living in infected districts, the symptoms become developed between the 10th and the 25th year. In four out of 149 such cases, the age at the commencement of the attack varied from four to six years; four patients were between 52 and 56, and two between 62 and 64 years. It is doubtful whether leprous symptoms have ever been observed in a new-born infant.

Taking into consideration the facts and arguments as stated in the preceding paragraphs, it would seem that heredity has a considerable share in the causation of leprosy, but that it fails to account for the terrible frequency of the disease. The prevalence of leprosy is mainly due to contagion.

In order to complete this account of the etiology of leprosy, some mention must be made of those conditions which appear to further the development and spread of the disease. Some of these predisposing causes have been invested with a much higher degree of importance than really belongs to them. Those which require notice are locality, climate, and rapid changes of temperature; deficient or unsuitable food; insanitary conditions of various kinds; the influence of previous diseases, etc.

1. *Locality and climate.*—The inhabitants of districts bordering on the sea have been regarded as more prone to be attacked than persons living inland, and the experience of Norway, Spain, Portugal, and of many parts of India, China, etc., seems to confirm this opinion. There are, however, many facts which point to an opposite conclusion. In various parts of the world the disease is even more prevalent hundreds of miles from the shore than it is on or near the coast. With regard to climate, the prevalence of the disease is little, if at all, influenced by any such conditions as temperature, moisture of air, rainfall, and the like, save in so far as they may impair the general health of the inhabitants, and render them more likely to be affected by injurious influences.

2. *Deficient or unsuitable food.*—It was only natural that in former times the cause of the disease should have been sought for in the diet of the sufferers. That this view is utterly without foundation is proved by the fact that leprosy occurs in some

countries and districts in which food is plentiful, and in many respects appropriate. The immoderate use of fish as food, of certain kinds of fish, and of salt and putrid fish, has been thought to be the cause of the disease, and this view has been adopted by Mr. Hutchinson. The development of leprosy has been ascribed by other authorities to the excessive use of pork. With regard to fish-diet, it is doubtless true that the food of Norwegian peasants and fishermen is often poor in quality and very indigestible; gastric catarrh and dyspepsia in various forms are very prevalent among these classes. Their diet consists of fish, and mainly of herrings, in a semi-rotten state, pickled in tainted brine; of other fish more or less decomposed, salted, dried, and always imperfectly cooked; of curdled sour milk, kept, perhaps, for weeks or months; of small quantities of potatoes with a little bread made of oatmeal; of broth made from the same flour, with a little salt meat or bacon from time to time—all such articles being often washed down by mouthfuls of so-called *aqua vitæ*. Added to all these defects is the utter indifference of the peasants as to the water they drink, and the vessels in which it is kept. The water is not only bad, but it is generally kept in a sort of cask, or in a hole made in the earth, and surrounded by impurities of various kinds, and pools of dirty water. But that such unwholesome food is not the cause of leprosy is proved by the fact that the fishermen and peasants on the north and south coasts of Norway, as badly fed as their compatriots on the west coast, are nearly, if not quite, exempt from the disease (Leloir). Leprosy is also unknown among the fishermen of Newfoundland, who live almost entirely upon fish.

With regard to the immoderate use of pork as a cause of leprosy, Dr. Hirsch quotes recent statements from physicians in Mexico, where leprosy is common and pork is a staple article of food. "There are many lepers who have never eaten pork, others who have partaken of it rarely, and still others who have lived on it to an excessive extent; but among all these the disease occurred with equal intensity. We conclude from this that the use of that article of diet has no influence whatsoever either upon the production of the disease or upon the severity of its type."

We may take another example, cited by Dr. Leloir, and contrast it with Norwegian experience. Cases of leprosy in the Riviera occur among persons dwelling in a very healthy country. The inhabitants are not exposed to cold; they are cleanly in their habits; they do not eat fish; but their diet consists almost exclusively of vegetables, fruits, flour, etc. It is thus evident that many of the causes and conditions to which leprosy has been attributed are not to be found in the Riviera. The patients are by no means invariably poor; one leprous girl had a marriage portion of 50,000 francs.

3. *Other insanitary conditions* may predispose individuals to become affected with leprosy, though they cannot of themselves give rise to the disease. Exposure to very severe weather, want of proper shelter, insufficient clothing and uncleanly habits of all kinds may be placed in this category. That they play only a very secondary part in the causation of leprosy is demonstrated by the fact that the disease may be absent when all the conditions co-exist. Thus in Terra del Fuego we find a combination of almost all possible insanitary conditions, and yet there are no cases of leprosy. Examples of the same character might easily be multiplied. It is, of course, admitted that in infected districts the disease is more apt to attack the necessitous classes than those who are

more favourably situated, though persons in good circumstances do not enjoy exemption.

4. With regard to the *effect of previous diseases* on the development of leprosy, all that can be said is that such disorders as syphilis, scurvy, tuberculosis, and malarious fevers, in so far as they impair the general health, adapt the individual, so to speak, for the reception of the virus. It is, however, impossible that any of these disorders can actually cause leprosy. Some authors have gone so far as to declare that the disease has sometimes been produced by fatigue, excitement, etc. In Norway, however, the population generally shows decided signs of vigour, and leprosy selects its victims from the strong as well as from the weak.

Leprosy is a contagious disease, and due to a specific virus. It is capable of being transmitted by parents to their offspring. Other alleged causes of leprosy are operative only so far as they impair the general health.

CHAPTER IV.

THE TREATMENT AND PREVENTION OF LEPROSY.

LEPROSY is an incurable disease; that is to say, it cannot be brought to an end by any form of treatment. It is true that in some very rare cases the morbid process appears to cease, but not until more or less serious damage has been effected. The march of the disease is arrested; but such results as paralyses and mutilations of various kinds are of course permanent.

It is not to be wondered at that many remedies have been tried with the hope of finding some specific, or at least some drug that would exercise a favourable influence upon the course of the disease. The list includes mercury, iodide and bromide of potassium, antimony, arsenic, phosphorus, bismuth, etc.; while among vegetable drugs, sarsaparilla, hydrocotyle asiatica, chaulmoogra, secale cornutum, anacardium (cashew nut), gurjun balsam, chrysarobin (goa powder), copaiba balsam, digitalis and many others have been tried, but all in vain. Salicylic acid, carbolic acid, and creasote (both given internally as well as applied to ulcers) have been lauded by some physicians, and, so far as our present knowledge extends, the use of these and of other antiseptics and parasiticides may be said to offer some prospect of success. In some cases, they certainly bring about a decided improvement in the local manifestations; and this is, at least, sufficient to show that medical science is not altogether helpless in the presence of this terrible disease.

With regard to the mineral remedies, the general statement holds good that all are useless, and some extremely mischievous. Mercury and iodine belong to the latter category; and each of these powerful drugs has been very extensively used. Mercury always does harm in cases of true leprosy; it readily produces salivation and ulceration of the mouth and throat in these patients. When, as not unfrequently happens, a leper contracts syphilis, mercury may perhaps be desirable. It should be given with the greatest caution, and in very small doses; it is less likely to do harm in cases of anæsthetic leprosy than in those of the pronounced tuberous type. Its alleged beneficial effects in cases of leprosy can be explained only by supposing that the diagnosis was incorrect, and that the patients were really suffering from syphilis. Iodine is almost equally injurious; Danielssen states that its preparations are liable to cause the symptoms to assume an acute form. A similar remark applies to the bromides.

Arsenic, antimony and phosphorus exercise little, if any, influence upon the course of the disease; in large doses, they would certainly prove injurious.

In a few cases, comparatively good results have followed the employment of the vegetable remedies above mentioned. Dr. Vandyke Carter and others speak highly of chaulmoogra oil (Oleum Gynocardiæ). All that can be said is that occasionally the local symptoms are much ameliorated under its use. It is given internally in doses of gr. xv and upwards, and likewise applied in the form of an ointment.

Gurjun balsam is another remedy of this class. An emulsion is made with an equal volume of lime-water, and this is used freely as a liniment and also given in doses of four drachms several times a day. The Norwegian physicians have given this drug an extensive trial, but without any decidedly good result. Dr. Bidenkap states that frictions with the liniment seemed to have a favourable influence on the diseased cutaneous nerves—about the same as that of massage.

Goa powder and its constituent, chrysophanic acid, have been especially recommended by Dr. Unna (*Monatshefte für Pract. Dermatologie,* July, 1885). He states that the external application of the drug, combined with the internal use of a preparation named ammonium sulphichthyolicum, will cure cases of incipient tuberous leprosy. His reports of two cases are certainly very encouraging. In Dr. Bidenkap's hands this treatment has perhaps done some good in one case, but has completely failed in several others.

According to Dr. Fleming,* Brigade Surgeon, Bengal Army, carbolic acid is a valuable remedy in cases that have not advanced beyond the first stages. He used as an application to the surface a mixture of carbolic acid and oil or glycerine (1 to 8 or more) and gave ♏j-iv. of the acid internally several times a day. Ten cases were thus treated, and most of them were decidedly improved. The internal administration did not seem to have any direct action upon the

---

* "Notes on the Carbolic Treatment of Leprosy," 1889. Reprinted from the *Indian Medical Gazette.*

disease, the progress being at much the same rate as when the acid was only employed externally.

Whatever estimate may be formed of the value of the remedies thus rapidly passed under review, the fact must always be borne in mind that, even in the absence of any special treatment, the course of leprosy is often interrupted by remissions, especially in the early stages. Not only may the morbid process come to a standstill, but a decided improvement may take place, and may progress so far that the patient appears to be almost, if not quite, free from the disease. A change of this character is a not very unfrequent result of removal from an infected district, and of attention to the general health. The improvement, however, in all but a small minority of cases, is not permanent; reappearance of the symptoms is the almost invariable rule. Hence the suspicion with which one must regard all accounts of the "cure" of leprosy; and especially those in which the patients have remained only a few months under observation. As a case in point, Dr. Hardy cites that of Dr. Lepine, who was said to have been "cured" by the use of hydrocotyle asiatica. The disease proved fatal in less than three years after the supposed cure.

Prof. Cornil, believing that leprosy is due to the presence of a microbe, endeavoured to discover another micro-organism, which would act as a *gendarme* and overpower or destroy the microbe. With this view he injected an infusion of jequirity under the skin of a leprous patient. The result, however, was by no means satisfactory. No change took place in the external manifestations, and some time afterwards the symptoms of mixed leprosy broke out in a very severe form. According to Dr. Leloir, Prof. Campana had a still more unfortunate experience in his endeavour to combat the leprosy bacillus. He inoculated two lepers with matter obtained from a case of erysipelas. The result was that the latter spread to nearly all the patients in the ward, while the leprous symptoms remained unaffected.

Attempts to cure the disease having proved unavailing, it is satisfactory to learn that much may often be done in the way of palliating many of the symptoms. Thus the neuralgic pains, which frequently torture the unfortunate patients to a degree almost indescribable, are sometimes considerably relieved by vapour baths, tepid baths, by cupping along the course of the affected nerve, and by salicylate of sodium administered internally. These remedies are frequently used in Norway. As an application to the tubers, and for the erythema, Dr. Bidenkap recommends the Goa powder in the form of an ointment. Massage sometimes produces good effects both on tuberous growths and on thickened nerves. Nerve-stretching has been tried for the relief of very severe pain, and it may be resorted to if everything else fails.

The lesions of the eye, which constitute a frequent and much dreaded complication of leprosy, and in the absence of treatment often lead to total blindness, can be much ameliorated by medical skill. Dr. Kaurin, for instance, often performs keratotomy in order to prevent the spread of the tubercles to the cornea. Danielssen recommends, for the same purpose, the application of caustics. Dr. Kaurin also performs various operations with the object of raising the lower eyelid, so that the eye can be partially closed and the tears prevented from running over the cheek. The importance of these operations may be gauged by the frequency with which affections of the eye occur among lepers. Out of 64 cases at Molde, 41 presented ocular lesions; 37 of these had both eyes affected, and six were quite blind (Leloir).

Amputation of the affected limb is sometimes performed, and with good results, when the neuralgic pains have become insupportable in spite of all remedies. Dr. Leloir records such a case, under the care of Dr. Kaurin at Molde, in 1881. The operation was followed by complete subsidence of the pain, and the wound healed satisfactorily. Dr. Leloir thinks that caustics of various kinds, and also the actual cautery, may occasionally be employed with advantage for the destruction of the tubercles. In his opinion tuberous leprosy is sometimes a purely local complaint, and he believes that the destruction or removal of the growths at their first appearance, and when only a few exist, might ward off general infection of the system. He cites another case of Dr. Kaurin's, in which the tubercles were confined to the left leg, converting it into a misshapen mass covered with ulcers. Amputation of the thigh was performed, with improvement of the general health, as the immediate result. During the succeeding nine months the patient showed no trace of leprosy.

I have discussed at some length the subject of treatment, in order to show that although no cure has as yet been discovered for leprosy, many of the more distressing symptoms can be much ameliorated by the aid of medicine and surgery. This fact admits of no dispute, and the lesson to be drawn from it surely is that lepers should not be neglected in the fashion which prevails in most of the infected countries, but should be admitted into special institutions, and subjected to kindly and careful treatment. As Dr. Leloir says, a leper ought not to be an object of horror or of neglect; he ought to inspire sympathy and devotion.

Before discussing the question of prophylaxis, a few remarks on some details of hygienic treatment will not be out of place. In all but very advanced cases, the patients should, whenever possible, be removed from an infected district into a healthy country, enjoying a temperate climate. In any case, they should be placed under as favourable hygienic conditions as circumstances will permit. The food should be nutritious, and non-stimulating in character, and consist mainly of meat, eggs, milk, and fresh vegetables. All indigestible articles, as salted meats, salt fish, etc., should be forbidden. Alcoholic drinks, if allowed at all, must be given in very small quantities. The skin should be kept as clean as possible; vapour baths and tepid baths, containing a little permanganate of potassium, carbolic acid, or thymol should be frequently employed. They act favourably on the skin, and on the patient's general health. Cold baths are not desirable.

When ulcers or sores exist, they should be kept very clean, and dressed with various antiseptic ointments and lotions. Ulceration of the mouth and throat requires gargles, powders (by insufflation) and fluid antiseptics and deodorants, applied by means of the spray-apparatus. Tonics of various kinds, and especially iron and quinine, are often useful. Sulphur waters taken internally and used for baths, are said to have produced good results. Any intercurrent symptoms must be treated according to their nature; diarrhœa is sometimes very troublesome, and requires astringents of various kinds. Tracheotomy is occasionally necessary in order to avert impending asphyxia.

The importance of all attempts to improve the general health of leprous patients cannot be overrated. Next in order comes the internal and external employment of antiparasitic remedies.

It now remains (1) to consider various measures that have been adopted in order to check the spread of leprosy; (2) to endeavour to estimate their real value, and (3) to point out the lessons to be deduced therefrom.

In the earliest times, and down to a comparatively modern date, there was no difference of opinion with regard to the contagiousness of leprosy and the measures required for preventing its spread. More or less rigorous isolation of the sufferers was enjoined by laws, to the non-observance of which severe penalties were attached. In most countries, lepers were expelled from their dwelling-places, and made to live apart beyond the gates of towns, in hospitals, or in "houses of separation." Prof. Marks tells us that "Jewish lepers were, under penalty of eighty stripes, forbidden to approach the mountain of the Temple; yet they were not rigidly confined to isolation, but were allowed to move about freely, and, in towns without walls, even allowed to enter Synagogues. It was of the utmost importance that they should, on the remotest suspicion, present themselves for inspection to competent authorities, such as the appointed priests, and should be pronounced clean only after repeated and most scrupulous examination. They had no right to complain of a personal restriction which was imposed in the interest of society as well as in their own; for society was freed from apprehension and danger, and they themselves from a distrust, which, even when unfounded, was sure to injure their social position. If declared to be infested with the evil, they were required to make themselves strikingly known at first glance; like mourners, they were to appear in public with rent garments, bare head and covered beard; thus signalized they would surely be shunned; but if anyone should inadvertently come near them, they were to warn him off by the loud wail, 'Unclean, Unclean!' They were even interred in a separate burial-ground."

An account has been given in a previous chapter (see page 7) of the discipline to which lepers were subjected in England and abroad during the middle ages. In some countries, strict isolation appears to have been practised; in others, lepers were allowed to move more or less freely about the country, but were compelled to adopt certain measures to prevent other persons from approaching them. Thus we are told that they were obliged to make a constant noise with a rattle, to wear two artificial hands of white wool, one tied on the breast, the other on the head, and to call attention to their presence in various other ways.

2. It is not possible to determine, in a manner approaching to accuracy, the real value of the preventive measures thus briefly alluded to. The fact remains that cases of leprosy became less and less frequent in Europe in the fifteenth and sixteenth centuries; and that the decline of the disease was in proportion to the rigour with which isolation was enforced upon the sufferers. Other causes, doubtless, co-operated in producing the effect. During the middle ages, and even at a much later date in some countries in Europe, the articles of food consumed by the people in general were for the most part of an unwholesome and innutritious character. Fresh meat was a luxury within the reach of comparatively few; salted provisions, both tough and indigestible, represented the animal portion of diet; fresh vegetables and fruits were scarce and often unobtainable, and even the bread was generally of a kind from which even the poorest would now turn away in disgust. The habitations and surroundings of the people presented many conditions in the highest degree favourable to the spread of epidemics; water was generally scarce and often bad; the arrangements for the disposal of excreta were of the rudest character.

Slowly, but surely, a progressive improvement took

place in many respects. The food of the poorer classes became more varied, more abundant, and more nutritious in character, and some advance was made in the art of cookery; while, owing to the increasing spread of commerce with other countries, bad harvests were no longer followed by wide-spread famine. Social conditions in general were thus rendered much more favourable than at any previous time, and it is highly probable that the disappearance of leprosy was in some measure due to the improvements thus briefly specified. The isolation of the sick was, however, the most potent factor.

The condition of Norway, as regards leprosy, furnishes abundant evidence of the value of isolation, and it is to this subject that I wish to call special attention. All the physicians, whom I met in Norway, were unanimous in the opinion that *segregation was the most important part of the treatment of leprosy*. I would refer to the figures given on page 13, and will here only repeat that the number of lepers in Norway has decreased by one-half in the course of thirty-three years. A still more rapid diminution may be expected to take place in future, for it was only in 1885 that a law was passed authorizing a forced seclusion of lepers.

Asylums for lepers were founded in Norway as far back as the thirteenth century; but even in comparatively recent times their purpose, as Dr. Bidenkap says, was not to restrain the spread of leprosy by infection (which has only of late been accepted by Norwegian physicians), but to treat the unfortunate patients and to prevent the hereditary transmission of the disease. In 1845 a law was proposed, aiming to prevent the marriage of lepers, but was rejected by the Parliament. Previous to 1885 there was no effective law compelling the lepers to come into the hospitals; but the majority either came voluntarily or were driven to do so by their poverty; for the local authorities would not relieve them, whereas the hospitals supplied all necessaries. In 1885 a law was passed that all lepers (not in asylums) should be isolated in their homes, and that failure to comply with this regulation was to be followed by their compulsory removal to those institutions. Isolation of a leper in his own house means that he must remain in one room specially marked off for him; he may, however, walk about in the open air in the company of his friends or others, but he must not go into any other room than the one appointed to him. The adoption of these measures was entirely due to the indefatigable activity of the Norwegian physicians. They have convinced their fellow countrymen that leprosy is contagious, and that isolation of the patients is the only efficacious measure for stamping out the disease. At the same time they are far from ignoring the good effects of improved sanitation, diet, etc. There is every reason for expecting that leprosy will become extinct in Norway in the course of a few decades.

Another example, of a very different character, enforces the lesson to be drawn from Norwegian experience. Let us examine the statistics of leprosy in an island in which isolation of the patients is not carried out.

According to Dr. Neisser, the island of Trinidad contained—

In 1805 ...   3 lepers in a population of 29,940.
,, 1813 ... 73   ,,   ,,   ,,   ,, 32,000.
,, 1878 ... 860   ,,   ,,   ,,   ,, 120,000.

Dr. Leloir states that in 1884 the number of lepers was 450 among a population of 180,000; but he had been assured by a resident physician, Dr. de Verteuille, that that number by no means indicated the real state of the case. His informant also laid special stress upon the increasing frequency of the disease among the white population. "Fifty years ago there were not more than three or four white families among whom a leper could be found." At the present time, Dr. de Verteuille knows of at least fifteen such families, and he believes that more could be discovered. This increase is attributable to the fact that, although an asylum exists, the patients enter and leave it just as they like. It now contains three whites (two of whom are Europeans); 97 Africans and creoles and 43 coolies. Compulsory isolation has never been put in force by the Government. A century ago, when colonization began, there were a few cases scattered about over the island. No precautions having been taken, the number has steadily increased; and the proportion to the population was far less fifty years ago than it is at the present time. The emancipation of the slaves in 1834 was followed by a flow of immigration from the neighbouring colonies and from India, and the new comers brought with them a certain number of lepers. In Curaçao, another West Indian island, where the Dutch Government has for the last 40 years strictly carried out prophylactic measures, the number of lepers has been kept down to ten or twelve.

Another instance, also cited by Dr. Leloir, is that of the Guianas. The territories bearing that name are three in number, and belong to England, Holland, and France respectively. The Dutch territory is between the other two, and the Government adopts preventive measures with the same vigour as in Curaçao. The number of lepers is much less than in the adjacent territories where no similar precautions are taken, and where the complaint is decidedly on the increase. A report, teaching the same lesson, comes from Madagascar. Dr. Davidson says that when isolation was practised the spread of the disease was arrested, and that when the law ceased to be enforced the number of lepers enormously increased.

It would be easy to multiply examples demonstrating the value of isolation; there is one which must not be omitted. In New Brunswick persons affected with leprosy do not communicate freely with the rest of the community after the existence of the disease has been fully ascertained. They are admitted into a Lazaretto, where their friends and acquaintances are allowed to visit them occasionally, under certain restrictions. "For some years past," Dr. Taché states, "the segregation has not been enforced by violent measures; but the exertions, particularly on the part of the clergy, to induce the sick to enter the Lazaretto have been unceasing, and the result has been that for many years all lepers, with only two exceptions, have resorted to the Lazaretto." This institution was first established in 1844; it is supported at the public expense, and the patients are under the care of Sisters of Charity, a chaplain, and a physician. In 1885 the Lazaretto contained twenty-two patients. Owing to strict precautionary measures and to the effective isolation, the diminution in the number of the patients has been steadily going on for some years. Relatively to the population the decrease is very considerable.

3. The lessons to be drawn from the facts thus briefly narrated are significant and unmistakable. To check the spread of leprosy two measures must be adopted—the sufferers must be isolated, and the sanitary condition of inhabitants of infected districts must be improved in every possible manner. With regard to isolation, we find that Norway is the only European country in which this method is carried out.

Here in England we are so happily situated that a leper is one of the rarest of prodigies, and becomes an object of universal interest and commiseration. In some of our colonies and in our Eastern empire familiarity with leprosy seems to have bred contempt. In Hindostan, at all events, the disease is regarded as an evil far beyond the capacity of an all-powerful Government to prevent. A former Viceroy is reported to have said that one might almost as readily undertake to rid India of its snakes as of its lepers. So long as this notion prevails, any serious effort is of course not to be looked for. India may perhaps some day be governed by a Viceroy whose vocabulary does not contain the word "impossible." The task of ridding India of leprosy would be one of enormous magnitude and difficulty, and would require years of patient labour for its accomplishment. Yet considering what has been done in India, and the marvellous excellence of its administration, it would be casting an undeserved stigma on the governing classes to declare that they are powerless to prevent the spread of this terrible disease. It is unnecessary to repeat the accounts, lately given by many Indian journals, of the so-called "leper nuisance." These are some of the statements, the truth of which is beyond question. In India, lepers are allowed to wander about wherever they please; in large towns they haunt the markets, tramway stations, and other places of public resort, they squat around tanks, performing their ablutions and dressing their sores; and in the city of Bombay they are wont to congregate close to schools where thousands of boys are educated. One might well ask, What more could be done to promote the spread of the disease? After describing the condition of lepers in Bombay, one Indian paper aptly remarks: "We seem to be reading rather of the insanitary foulness of a mediæval city where medical science was still in its infancy, and men's conceptions of the duties and responsibilities of civic government still rudimentary, than of the state of things in a great city of the nineteenth century British empire."

The Indian Government has, however, done something; it has passed a resolution that for the present, at all events, it is impossible to do more than encourage the grant of medical and charitable relief in voluntary hospitals and leper-asylums. We are also told that instructions have been issued to district officers to endeavour to provide asylums for lepers, and that leave has been granted to employ for this purpose funds given for the support of dispensaries and other charitable objects. In the opinion of those well qualified to judge, steps of this character will prove to be almost if not quite inoperative to procure isolation of the sick and arrest the spread of the disease. There will be no power to compel lepers to reside in certain places, or to remain in asylums any longer than they choose. It is in vain to expect any good results from such measures as these. The leprosy question in India will have to be grappled with some day, and it will become more and more difficult as time goes on. Our knowledge of the disease is doubtless imperfect, but we are fully cognizant of its horrible character, and of the means by which alone its spread can be arrested. Compulsory isolation in suitable buildings and under proper care is urgently demanded in the interests not only of the general community, but of the sufferers themselves. If leprosy cannot be cured, some of the more distressing symptoms can certainly be alleviated.

INDEX.

A.

Africa, Leprosy in, 18.
America, United States of, Leprosy in, 20.
Anæsthetic leprosy, 31.
Antiparasitic treatment of leprosy, 76, 78.
Australia, Leprosy in, 18.

B.

Bacilli of leprosy, 48.
Bennett, Sir Risdon, on the leprosy of the Bible, 3.
Brazil, Leprosy in, 21.

C.

Canada, Leprosy in, 20.
Cape of Good Hope, Leprosy at the, 18.
Carbolic acid in treatment of leprosy, 78.
Cause of leprosy, 48.
Causes of death in leprosy, 43.
Causes, Predisposing, of leprosy, 69.
Chaulmoogra oil for leprosy, 77.
China, Leprosy in, 16.
Climate as a cause of leprosy, 70.
Contagiousness of leprosy, Proofs of, 54.
Curaçoa, Leprosy in, 91
Cures of leprosy, 79.
Cutaneous leprosy, 23.

D.

Definition of leprosy, 1.
Diagnosis of leprosy, 44.
Diet as a cause of leprosy, 70.
Disappearance of leprosy from British Isles, 9.
Disease, Previous, as a cause of leprosy, 74.

E.

England, Leprosy in, 7.
Eye, Affections of the, in leprosy, 36, 81.

F.

Food, Deficient or improper, as a cause of leprosy, 70.
Forms of leprosy, 23.
France, Leprosy in, 15.

G.

Geographical distribution of leprosy, 12.
Goa powder in leprosy, 78.
Greece, Leprosy in, 15.
Guianas, The, leprosy in, 92.
Gurjun balsam in leprosy, 77.

H.

Hereditary transmission of leprosy, 65.
Hindostan, Leprosy in, 16, 94.
Hirsch, Dr., on contagion of leprosy, 63.
Hygienic treatment of leprosy, 83.

I.

Incubation of leprosy, 62.
Inoculation of leprous matter, 57.

Iodine in the treatment of leprosy, 76.
Insanitary conditions as causes of leprosy, 73.
Isolation of leprous patients, 85.

J.

Japan, Leprosy in, 16.
Jews, Leprosy among the, 2, 85.

K.

Kaurin, Dr. Ed., on leprosy in Norway, 13, 41, 65, 81.

L.

Leloir, Dr., on contagiousness of leprosy, 68; geographical distribution of leprosy, 21; history, 11; inoculation of leprous matter, 58; leprosy in Norway, 14; in Trinidad, 90.

Leprosy, Causes of, 48; diagnosis of, 44; duration of life in, 40; earliest accounts of, 2; forms of, 23; incubation of, 62; "mixed," 40; morbid anatomy of, 47; mutilations due to, 35; paralyses in, 33; prevention of, 84; prognosis of, 42; symptoms of, 23; treatment of, 75.

Locality as a cause of leprosy, 70.

M.

Marks, Prof., on leprosy among the Jews, 85.
Mercury in the treatment of leprosy, 76.
Mexico, Leprosy in, 21.
Middle ages, Leprosy in the, 6.
Morbid anatomy of leprosy, 47.
Mutilations due to leprosy, 35.

N.

Neisser, Prof., on the leprosy bacillus, 48.
New Brunswick, Leprosy in, 92.
New Zealand, Leprosy in, 17.
Norway, Leprosy in, 12, 41, 81, 88.
Norwegian peasants, Diet of, 71

O.

Oceania, Leprosy in, 19.

P.

Paralysis due to leprosy, 33.
Pemphigus as a symptom of leprosy, 32.
Prevention of leprosy, 87.

R.

Russia, Leprosy in, 15.

S.

Sandwich Isles, Leprosy in, 11, 19, 57.
Simpson, Sir J., on leprosy, 7.
Spain, Leprosy in, 15.
Sweden, Leprosy in, 14.

T.

Trinidad, Leprosy in, 21, 90.
Trophic disorders in leprosy, 32.
Tuberous leprosy, 23.

U.

Ulcers in leprosy, 26.

W.

West Indies, Leprosy in, 21.

www.ingramcontent.com/pod-product-compliance
Lightning Source LLC
Chambersburg PA
CBHW031411160426
43196CB00007B/972